I0479195

CHILD HEALTH MANAGEMENT

The Ultimate Steps On How To Successfully Manage Any Child's Health

Ashley Brains

Copyright © 2023 by Ashley Brains

All rights reserved. No part of this book may be reproduced in any form or by any electronic or mechanical means, including information storage and retrieval systems, without written permission from the publisher or author, except in the case of a reviewer, who may quote brief passages in a review.

This book is a work of nonfiction. Any resemblance to persons, living or dead, or events is entirely coincidental.

Table of Contents

Introduction

John and Sarah had been married for almost a year when they welcomed their first child, a little girl they named Abigail. As first-time parents, they had a lot to learn about child health management.

John and Sarah knew it was important to keep their daughter healthy, so they made sure to keep up with all of her doctor's appointments and vaccinations. They also took the time to learn about nutrition and the importance of a balanced diet. They made sure Abigail was eating nutritious foods and avoiding processed and sugary snacks.

John and Sarah also took the time to create a safe environment for Abigail. They made sure her crib was up to safety standards and that all of her toys were non-toxic. They also taught her about safety, such as never crossing the street without an adult and always wearing a helmet when riding her bike.

John and Sarah also made sure to monitor Abigail's physical activity. They encouraged her to get outside and play, but also made sure she was getting enough rest. They regularly monitored her sleep and made sure she was getting the recommended amount of sleep for her age.

John and Sarah were also careful to keep an eye on Abigail's mental health. They made sure to spend quality time with her each day, talking and playing games. They kept her social life balanced, as well, making sure she had a good mix of playdates and time alone.

John and Sarah were proud of the job they were doing with Abigail's health management. They felt confident that they were giving her the best possible start in life.

Child health is a major concern for parents, caregivers, and the medical community alike. Ensuring that children receive proper nutrition, exercise, and medical care is essential to their physical, mental, and emotional wellbeing. Good child health is the foundation for a successful future and the key to preventing many health problems in adulthood. It is important to be aware of the health risks associated with child development and to take steps to ensure that children receive the best possible care and support. This includes providing access to health services, promoting healthy eating habits, and teaching children how to take care of their physical and mental health.

The health of children is a major concern for parents and healthcare professionals alike. Children face a variety of physical, mental, and emotional health issues that can have long-term implications for their development. Physical health issues such as obesity, asthma, allergies, and chronic illnesses can have an impact on a child's ability to participate in physical activities, socialize with peers, and perform well in school. Mental health issues such as depression, anxiety, and Attention Deficit Hyperactivity Disorder (ADHD) can have an impact on a child's ability to learn, interact with peers, and manage stress. Furthermore, emotional health issues such as bullying, abuse, and neglect can have an even greater impact on a child's development. It is important for parents, healthcare professionals, and educators to recognize and address these issues as early as possible to ensure that children have the best chance at leading healthy, successful lives.

Child health management is an important part of ensuring that children grow into healthy and productive adults. It involves monitoring and promoting the physical, psychological, and social well-being of children, as well as providing necessary medical care. This includes preventive and curative strategies such as proper nutrition, physical activities, immunizations, regular check-ups, and early detection and treatment of any health problems. Parents and caregivers play a vital role in child health management, as they are the primary source of support and guidance. Other professionals such as pediatricians, nurses, and social service workers also have an important role in providing health services to children. With the right resources and support, children can reach their full potential and lead healthy and happy lives.

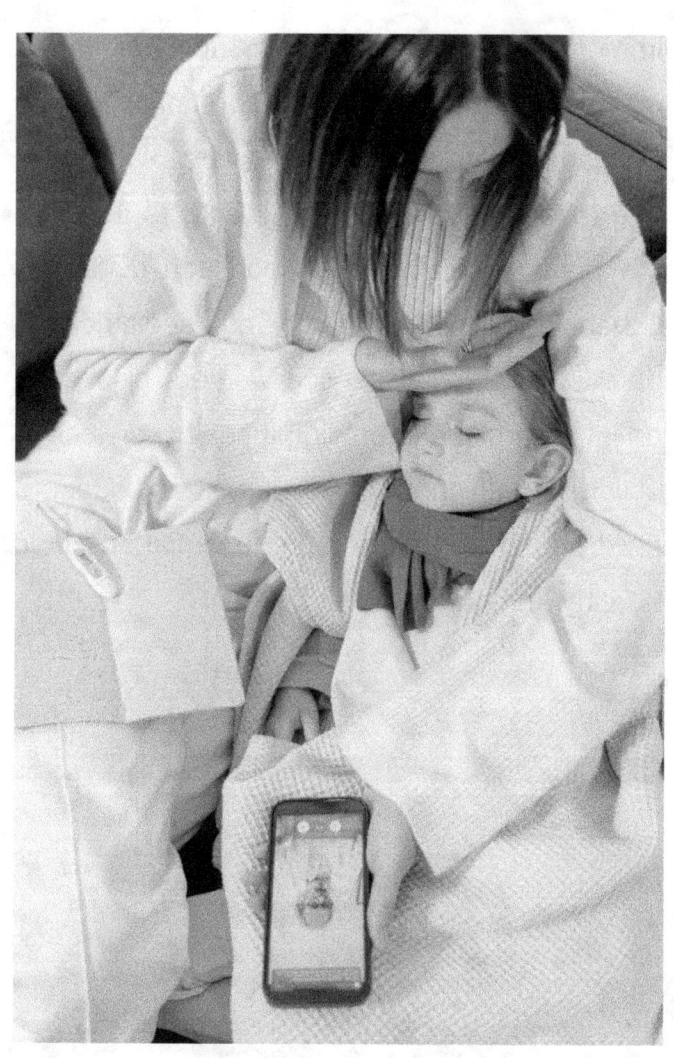

Chapter 1: The Beginning

Child health management is a critical part of any parent's responsibility. It is important for parents to understand how to best care for their children and ensure that they are reaching their full potential. This guide will provide an overview of the basics of child health management, from nutrition and physical activity, to immunizations and common illnesses.

Nutrition: Good nutrition is essential for children's growth and development. It is important to ensure that children get enough of the right kinds of foods, including fruits, vegetables, grains, dairy products, and protein. Parents should also limit their child's intake of sugary and processed foods, as these can contribute to obesity and other health problems.

Physical Activity: Regular physical activity is important for children's physical and emotional health. Encourage your child to participate in activities such as running, jumping, swimming, and biking. Set aside time each day for your child to be active, and make it fun.

Immunizations: Immunizations are necessary to protect children from serious diseases. It is important to make sure that your child is up to date on all of their immunizations.

Common Illnesses: It is important for parents to know the signs and symptoms of common illnesses, such as colds, flu, and stomach bugs. If your child is showing signs of illness, it is important to seek medical attention.

Child health management is an essential part of parenting. It is important to ensure that your child is receiving proper nutrition, physical activity, immunizations, and medical care. By following these tips, you can help ensure that your child is healthy and happy.

Prenatal Care

Parental care is an important factor in child health management. Parents are responsible for providing the basic needs of their children, including food, shelter, and clothing. Parents also have to ensure that their children receive regular medical care and vaccinations to help protect them from disease. Additionally, parents need to monitor their children's health, growth, and development, provide them with emotional and social support, and help them develop healthy habits.

Parents should be involved in all aspects of their child's health care, including visits to the pediatrician, monitoring of growth and development, and communication with health care providers. This can help parents stay informed about their child's health and track their progress. Parents should also discuss their child's health with their pediatrician and learn about any health concerns or needs that their child may have.

In addition to providing basic needs and medical care, parents can help their children stay active and healthy. This includes encouraging physical activities, such as playing outdoors or participating in sports, as well as providing healthy meals and snacks and limiting sugary, fatty, and processed foods. Parents should also help their children develop healthy habits, such as brushing their teeth and washing their hands regularly. Finally, parents should provide emotional and social support to their children, such as praising them for their accomplishments and helping them develop strong self-esteem.

Parental care is an essential part of child health management. Parents should be involved in their child's health care, help their children stay physically and emotionally healthy, and provide emotional and social support. Doing so can help children grow up to be healthy and happy adults.

Maternal and Fetal Health

Maternal and fetal health are integral components of child health management. Healthy mothers and babies are essential for a safe and successful pregnancy, birth, and postpartum period. As such, maternal and fetal health should be a priority in any health care system.

Maternal health is an important factor in the health and wellbeing of both mother and baby. During the prenatal period, it is important for mothers to receive proper care, nutrition, and exercise to ensure their own well-being, as well as the health of their unborn child. Regular visits with a health care provider are essential to monitor the mother's health and the development of the baby.

Fetal health is also an important consideration in child health management. It is essential that the unborn baby is monitored throughout the pregnancy to ensure it is growing and developing properly. Regular ultrasound scans can provide information about the baby's size and development, as well as detect any potential abnormalities. Regular checkups with a health care provider are important to monitor the baby's growth and development, and to ensure that any potential problems are addressed quickly.

During the postpartum period, it is important for the mother and baby to receive the necessary care to ensure their continued health and wellbeing. The mother should receive proper nutrition and exercise, as well as support from family and friends. The baby should receive regular checkups to monitor its growth and development, and should receive necessary vaccinations and treatments.

Maternal and fetal health are essential for the health and wellbeing of both mother and baby. It is important that the mother receives the necessary care, nutrition, and exercise during the prenatal period, and that the unborn baby is monitored throughout the pregnancy to ensure its health and development. Additionally, both the mother and baby should receive proper care during the postpartum period to ensure their continued health and wellbeing. With proper care and monitoring, mothers and babies can have a safe and successful pregnancy, birth, and postpartum period.

Nutrition and Supplements During Pregnancy

Good nutrition is essential for a healthy pregnancy and the proper development of a baby. Eating a balanced diet and taking prenatal vitamins can help ensure that both mother and baby are getting all the necessary nutrients. During pregnancy, women should focus on eating nutrient-dense foods, such as fruits and vegetables, whole grains, lean proteins, and low-fat dairy products. They should also limit their intake of processed foods, sugar, and saturated fats.

Supplements can also play an important role in providing additional nutrients to pregnant women. The most important supplements for pregnant women are folate, iron, and calcium. Folate helps prevent neural tube defects in the baby and helps protect the mother from anemia during pregnancy. Iron helps prevent anemia and is important for the baby's development. Calcium is an essential mineral necessary in making and building effective bones and teeth.

In addition to these three essential supplements, pregnant women may also benefit from taking a daily multivitamin. A multivitamin can help ensure that a woman is getting all the necessary vitamins and minerals she needs during pregnancy.

It is important to talk to a doctor before taking any supplements during pregnancy. Some supplements, such as fish oil, may not be safe for pregnant women, while others may be beneficial. A doctor can help determine which supplements are safe for a pregnant woman to take.

Good nutrition and supplements are essential for a healthy pregnancy and the proper development of a baby. Eating a balanced diet, taking prenatal vitamins, and talking to a doctor about any additional supplements can help ensure that both mother and baby are getting all the necessary nutrients during pregnancy.

Chapter 2: The Health and Development of a Child

When thinking about the health of a child, it's important to consider both their physical and mental wellbeing. It's essential that parents provide their children with the tools they need to maintain their health and foster a positive outlook on life.

Physical Health

Physical health is an important part of any child's life. Ensuring that your child is getting enough exercise and eating right is key to their physical health. Exercise should be incorporated into their daily routine, and meals should include a variety of healthy food choices. Parents should also ensure that their children are getting appropriate amounts of sleep.

Mental Health

It's important to know that the mental health of a child is crucial. It's essential that you provide your child with a supportive and loving environment. Talk with them about their thoughts and feelings and provide them with a safe space to express themselves. Encourage them to maintain positive relationships with their friends and family.

Pediatrics

Pediatrics is a specialty in medicine that deals with the medical care of infants exhaustively. It is concerned with promoting children's physical, mental, and social health and well-being. Pediatricians provide preventive care, diagnose and treat illnesses, and monitor the health of children.

Pediatricians are trained to recognize, diagnose, and treat common childhood illnesses, injuries, and developmental delays. They also provide guidance on how to maintain children's health through proper nutrition, hygiene, and physical activity. Pediatricians also provide preventive care, such as immunizations and regular checkups, to help children maintain their health.

The goals of pediatric care are to prevent illness and injury, diagnose and treat acute and chronic medical conditions, and promote a healthy lifestyle. Pediatricians relate closely with parents to ensure that infants and children get the best health care. They also provide education and counseling on topics such as nutrition, growth and development, and behavior.

Pediatricians are important members of the health care team, providing expertise on how to best care for children. They work closely with other health care providers, such as primary care physicians, nurses, and specialists, to ensure that children receive the best possible care. Pediatricians also provide support to families, helping them to understand and cope with their child's illness or developmental delay.

Pediatric care is an important part of child health management. Pediatricians provide preventive care, diagnose and treat illnesses, and monitor the health of children. They also provide education and counseling on topics such as nutrition, growth and development, and behavior. By working closely with parents and other health care providers, pediatricians help children stay healthy and reach their full potential.

Child Development

Child development is an incredibly important aspect of children's health and wellbeing. It refers to the physical, emotional, cognitive and social changes that occur in children as they grow and mature. As children grow, they face a variety of challenges and opportunities that can affect their development. It is important for parents, health professionals, and educators to ensure that children are receiving the necessary support and guidance to help them reach their full potential.

Physical Development

Physical development refers to the growth and development of the body's muscles, bones, and organs, as well as its size and shape.

Physical development in children is marked by milestones, such as crawling, walking, and talking. It is important for children to have regular physical activity to support healthy growth and development. Parents should ensure that their children are getting enough exercise to promote healthy physical development.

Emotional Development

Emotional development involves the development of a child's ability to recognize and express emotions, as well as regulate their emotions in a healthy way. Emotional development is important for a child's overall wellbeing, and it is essential for the development of their social, cognitive, and physical skills. Parents can help support their children's emotional development by providing them with a safe and secure environment where they can express their feelings and learn how to manage their emotions.

Cognitive Development

Cognitive development refers to the development of a child's thinking and reasoning skills. Cognitive development includes a child's ability to process and understand information, problem solve, and learn new skills. It is important for parents to provide children with stimulating activities that encourage learning and problem solving. This can include activities such as reading, playing games, and doing puzzles.

Social Development

Social development involves the development of a child's ability to interact with others, form relationships, and understand the behavior of others. Social development is essential for children to learn how to cooperate with others and develop healthy relationships. Parents can help support their children's social development by providing them with plenty of opportunities to play and interact with other children.

Overall, child development is an incredibly important aspect of a child's health and wellbeing. It is important for parents, health professionals, and educators to support children's physical, emotional, cognitive, and social development to help them reach their full potential.

Vaccinations and Immunizations

Vaccination and immunization are two of the most important aspects of child health management. Vaccines help to protect children from serious diseases, while immunization helps to ensure that children are not exposed to diseases for which they have not been vaccinated.

Vaccines work by introducing a weakened or killed form of a disease-causing microorganism into the body. This helps the body to recognize and fight off a specific infection if the person is later exposed to it. Vaccines are typically administered through shots and have been proven to be safe and effective in preventing a wide range of infectious diseases. Examples of common childhood vaccinations include the measles, mumps, and rubella (MMR) vaccine; the diphtheria, tetanus, and pertussis (DTaP) vaccine; the varicella (chickenpox) vaccine; and the hepatitis B vaccine.

Immunization is the process of stimulating the body's immune system to recognize and respond to a particular antigen. This can be done through a variety of methods, including exposure to a weakened or killed form of the disease-causing organism, or through injection of a substance containing the antigen. Immunization is important for protecting children from diseases for which they have not been vaccinated.

Vaccination and immunization are both essential components of child health management. Vaccines help to protect children from serious diseases, while immunization helps to ensure that children are not exposed to diseases for which they have not been vaccinated. It is important for parents and caregivers to ensure that their children receive the recommended vaccinations and immunizations on schedule in order to protect their health.

Screening and Diagnostics

Screening and diagnostics are two important components of child health management. Screening is the process of looking for potential health problems in seemingly healthy children, while diagnostics involves the use of tests and other procedures to accurately identify and diagnose a health condition.

Screening is important because it allows for early detection of health problems, which can be treated more successfully when discovered early. Examples of screenings for children include vision and hearing tests, growth and developmental assessments, as well as tests for infectious diseases, such as measles and tuberculosis.

Diagnostics is used to confirm a diagnosis and monitor the progression of a health condition. Examples of diagnostic tests include blood tests, urine tests, imaging tests (including X-rays and ultrasounds), and genetic tests.

Both screening and diagnostics are essential in child health management. Screening helps to detect health problems early, while diagnostics confirms the diagnosis and aids in the treatment and management of health conditions. It is important that parents and doctors work together to ensure that children receive the necessary screenings and tests in order to maintain their health. Regular visits to the doctor, as well as preventive care, will help to ensure that children receive the best possible health care.

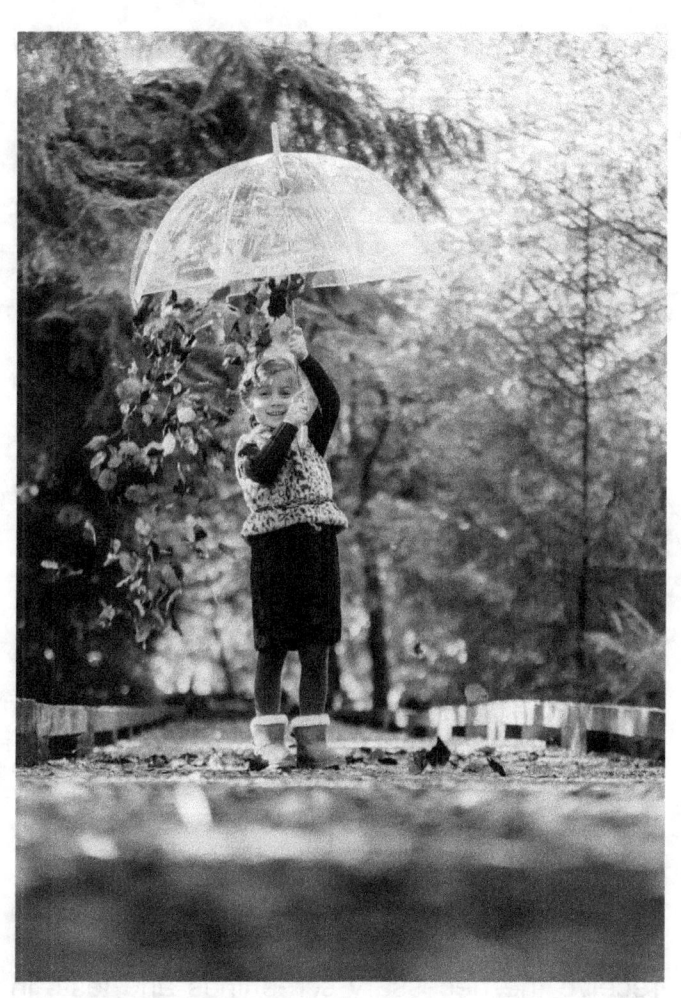

Chapter 3: Health Emergency

Child health management is an important part of any family's health care plan. Many parents worry about their child's health and how to make sure their child gets the best care available. It's important for parents to know what to do in case of a health emergency. Knowing the risks and how to respond can save a child's life.

First, it's important to be prepared for a health emergency. Every parent should know the basics of first aid and CPR to be able to respond appropriately in an emergency situation. Knowing the symptoms of common childhood illnesses and injuries is also essential. Keeping a list of important numbers and contact information, such as the family doctor and local hospital, can also help in an emergency.

Second, parents should be alert to changes in their child's health. This includes regularly monitoring their child's temperature, pulse and respiration rate. It's also important to watch for unusual behavior or physical symptoms that could indicate a medical emergency.

Third, parents should be aware of the warning signs of a health emergency. These can include difficulty breathing, sudden onset of a fever, loss of consciousness, chest pain, severe abdominal pain, severe headache or vomiting, rash, confusion or difficulty speaking, or a seizure. If any of these signs occur, parents should seek medical attention immediately.

Finally, it's important for parents to be aware of the various health emergencies that can affect children. These can include allergies, asthma, diabetes, poisoning, head injuries, fevers, seizures, and more. Knowing how to respond in each of these situations is essential for the safety of the child.

It's essential for parents to be aware of the risks and know how to respond in a health emergency. Being prepared and knowing the warning signs can help save a child's life in an emergency.

Recognizing Signs of Illness

Recognising the signs of illness in children is an important part of managing their health. It is important to be aware of any changes in your child's behaviour, so that you can take action if necessary. Early diagnosis and treatment can prevent serious health problems from developing.

One of the first signs of illness in children may be changes in their behaviour. Your child may seem more irritable or lethargic than usual. They may also be more clingy and have difficulty sleeping. Other signs of illness can include a decrease in appetite, coughing, sneezing, and fever. If your child is complaining of pain, it is important to take them to a doctor to be checked out.

It is also important to look out for physical changes that may indicate a health problem. For example, if your child has a rash, blotchy skin, or yellowing of the eyes or skin, this could be a sign of a more serious underlying health problem. If your child has a fever, it is important to take their temperature regularly to track any changes in their health.

When it comes to recognizing signs of illness, it is important to be aware of any changes in your child's routine. If your child is missing school or not engaging in activities they normally enjoy, this could be a sign that something is wrong. It is also important to be aware of any changes in your child's weight or appetite.

It is important to seek medical advice if you have any concerns about your child's health. A doctor can assess your child's symptoms and provide an accurate diagnosis and treatment plan. Early diagnosis and treatment can help to prevent any further health problems from developing.

Recognising the signs of illness in children is an important part of managing their health. It is important to be aware of any changes in your child's behaviour and physical appearance, so that action can be taken if necessary. If you have any concerns about your child's health, it is important to seek medical advice. Early diagnosis and treatment can help to prevent any further health problems from developing.

Emergency Care and Treatment

When it comes to child health, emergency situations can arise quickly and without warning. It is essential that parents and caregivers are aware of how to recognize an emergency as well as how to respond. Knowing the appropriate emergency care and treatment for children can help to ensure that they receive the right care in the most appropriate setting.

First and foremost, it is important to recognize the signs and symptoms of a medical emergency. These can include chest pain, difficulty breathing, uncontrolled bleeding, severe burns, sudden changes in mental status, or severe pain. If any of these symptoms are observed, it is important to seek medical help immediately. Do not try to diagnose the condition or administer treatment without medical assistance.

In the event of an emergency, it is important to stay calm and act quickly. Call 911 or your local emergency number for assistance. Provide the operator with as much information as possible about the child's condition and be prepared to follow any instructions given. In some cases, the operator may advise you to bring the child to the nearest emergency room or trauma center.

If you are able to transport the child to the hospital, it is important to remember to bring any relevant medical history, including medications that the child is taking. It is also important to bring along any insurance information and identification documents. If possible, have another adult accompany you to provide additional support.

Once at the hospital, the medical team will assess the child's condition and provide the appropriate emergency care and treatment. Depending on the severity of the situation, the child may need to be admitted to the hospital for further care. In some cases, the child may need to be transferred to a larger hospital or specialty care center.

It is important to remember that the goal of emergency care and treatment is to stabilize the child's condition and provide the necessary medical attention. Depending on the situation, the child may need to remain in the hospital for a few days or weeks. During this time, parents and caregivers should make sure to communicate with the medical team and keep updated on the child's progress.

By being aware of the appropriate emergency care and treatment for child health management, parents and caregivers can help ensure that their child receives the best possible care. In the event of an emergency, it is important to remain calm and take the necessary steps to get the child the help they need.

Chapter 4

Mental and Behavioral Health

Mental and behavioral health is an important factor in the overall health and development of children. The physical and emotional well-being of a child are inextricably linked, and mental and behavioral health must be addressed in order to ensure the optimal health of a child. Mental and behavioral health problems can range from mild to severe and can have a significant impact on a child's development and well-being.

Child health management is the practice of monitoring, diagnosing, and treating children's physical and mental health. This includes assessing a child's overall health, identifying and diagnosing mental and behavioral health issues, and developing a plan of care that meets the needs of the individual child. It also involves providing support and resources to parents and caregivers to ensure they are equipped to support their child's health.

The first step in child health management is to recognize the signs and symptoms of mental and behavioral health issues. These can range from anxiety and depression to more serious conditions such as autism or attention-deficit/hyperactivity disorder (ADHD). It is important to be aware of these signs and symptoms and to identify them early so that appropriate interventions can be provided.

The next step is to diagnose the mental and behavioral health issue. This may involve a combination of medical tests, psychological assessments, and behavioral observations. Once the diagnosis is made, a treatment plan can be developed. This may include psychotherapy, medication, and lifestyle changes, as well as other interventions.

In addition to these interventions, it is important to provide families with resources and support to help them manage their child's mental and behavioral health. This may include access to mental health professionals, support groups, and educational materials. It is also important to provide parents with information about how to talk to their child about mental and behavioral health issues and how to help them manage their emotions and behaviors.

Child health management is an important part of caring for children. It is important to recognize the signs and symptoms of mental and behavioral health issues and to provide the necessary resources and support to ensure that children receive the care they need to lead healthy and productive lives.

Promoting Positive Mental Health

Mental health is an integral part of overall health and wellbeing, and it is important to pay attention to positive mental health in children. It is essential to promote positive mental health in children to ensure they have a strong foundation for good physical and emotional health.

Children who have positive mental health are better able to cope with stress, build relationships, and make healthy decisions. Encouraging positive mental health in children can help them develop self-esteem, resilience, and healthy coping skills.

Parents and caregivers can promote positive mental health in children by creating a safe and supportive home environment, modeling healthy behaviors, and helping children develop positive coping skills. Here are some tips on how to promote positive mental health in children:

• **Encourage healthy eating habits:** It is important to ensure that children are eating balanced meals, getting enough sleep, and engaging in physical activity. All of these activities help to promote positive mental health and can support children in developing healthy habits.

• **Model positive behavior:** Parents and caregivers should model positive behavior and good mental health practices. This includes being mindful of how you communicate with your children and setting a good example of how to handle stress and difficult emotions.

• **Connect with your child:** Spend quality time with your child and create a safe and supportive environment. Take an interest in your child's activities and show them that you care. This can help to strengthen your relationship and promote positive mental health.

• **Support your child:** Offer emotional support to your child and help them to build successful relationships with others. Show them that you are available to talk and listen if they have any worries or concerns.

• **Encourage positive coping skills:** Help your child to develop healthy coping skills such as problem-solving, relaxation techniques, and managing emotions. It can also be beneficial to help your child find activities or hobbies that they enjoy, as this can help them manage stress.

By promoting positive mental health in children, you can help to ensure that they have a strong foundation for long-term physical and emotional wellbeing. By following the tips outlined above, you can help your children to develop healthy habits and build resilience.

Recognizing and Treating Mental Health Concerns

Recognizing and treating mental health concerns in children is essential in order to help them cope with the challenges they face in life. Here are some strategies for recognizing and treating mental health concerns in children:

• **Talk to your child:** Talking to your child is one of the best ways to recognize and address mental health concerns. Ask your child how they are feeling, and listen to what they have to say. Encourage your child to express their emotions and provide a safe environment for them to do so.

• **Seek professional help:** If you are concerned about your child's mental health, consider seeking professional help from a mental health professional. A mental health professional can provide assessment, diagnosis, and treatment for mental health concerns.

• **Learn about mental health:** Educate yourself about mental health and how to recognize and treat mental health concerns in children. This can help you better understand your child's condition and provide more effective care.

• **Focus on positive coping skills:** Help your child develop positive coping skills to manage their mental health condition. Encourage them to engage in healthy activities, such as exercise, spending time with friends and family, and participating in hobbies

Chapter 5

Nutrition and Physical Activity

Proper nutrition and diet are important for a child's health, growth and development. Eating healthy foods and staying active helps children build strong bones and muscles, fight infections and maintain a healthy weight.

Nutrition and dietary guidelines for child health management are important to ensure that children are getting the essential nutrients they need for healthy growth and development. These guidelines can help parents, caregivers and health professionals create an optimal nutrition plan for children.

Here are a few nutrition and dietary guidelines to follow when managing a child's health:

1. Eat a variety of foods: Advice children to eat different kind of foods from the classes of food. This helps ensure that they are getting all the essential nutrients they need for healthy growth and development

2. Limit processed foods: Processed foods contains high sugar and salt composition which is unhealthy for children.

3. Encourage physical activity: Physical activity is important for a child's health, growth, and development. It helps maintain a healthy weight, builds strong bones and muscles, and boosts mental health.

4. Drink plenty of water. Water is essential for a child's health and should be consumed throughout the day.

5. Limit added sugars: Added sugars are often found in processed and junk foods.

These should be in a small amount in the child's diet.

6. Limit salt, saturated fats, and trans fats: These ingredients are often found in processed, fried, and fast foods. They should in a very small amount in the child's diet.

7. Encourage healthy snacking: Healthy snacks can help provide essential nutrients to a child's diet. Good snack options include whole-grain crackers with cheese, cut-up fruits and vegetables, yogurt, and nuts.

By following these nutrition and dietary guidelines, parents and caregivers can help children maintain a healthy weight, fight infections, and grow and develop properly. It is important to remember that every child's nutritional needs are different and that individualized nutrition plans should be created for each child to ensure their optimal health.

Physical Activity and Exercise

Physical activity and exercise are essential components of any health plan for children. Regular physical activity and exercise can help children build strong bones and muscles, improve cardiovascular health, and improve overall health and well-being.

Physical activity and exercise can help children maintain a healthy weight, reduce the risk of obesity, and reduce the risk of developing chronic diseases such as heart disease, diabetes, and depression. Children should engage in at least 60 minutes of physical activity each day to support their overall health. Physical activity can include any activity that gets the body moving, such as running, playing sports, dancing, or walking. Exercise is a form of physical activity that is designed to improve strength, flexibility, and endurance.

Physical activity and exercise are important for children's mental health and development. Regular physical activity can help children stay focused, improve concentration, and reduce stress and anxiety. Exercise can also help children develop important social skills, such as teamwork and communication.

Parents and caregivers can help children stay active by encouraging them to participate in physical activities and exercise. It is important for parents and caregivers to ensure that children are engaging in safe physical activity and exercise. This includes providing appropriate equipment and supervision, and ensuring that children are engaging in appropriate activities for their age and skill level.

Physical activity and exercise can also be fun and enjoyable for children. Parents and caregivers should encourage children to find activities that they enjoy, and to find ways to make physical activity and exercise part of their daily routine.

Physical activity and exercise are important for children's health and development. By encouraging children to participate in regular physical activity and exercise, parents and caregivers can help children build strong, healthy bodies, and support their overall health and wellbeing.

Conclusion

The conclusion of child health management is that it is essential for the well-being of children. Taking the time to assess, monitor, and address any health issues that may arise will ensure that children stay as healthy as possible. Parents and caregivers should be familiar with resources available to them to help address any health concerns that may arise. Additionally, they should provide their children with a balanced diet, regular exercise, and mental stimulation to promote strong physical and mental health. It is also important to ensure that vaccinations and screenings are up-to-date. With the right care and attention, children can have the best chance of leading long and healthy lives.

www.ingramcontent.com/pod-product-compliance
Lightning Source LLC
Chambersburg PA
CBHW081540220526
45467CB00010B/3270